Table of Contents

Chapter 1

Another year has passed and like an unconscious ritual, many of us make a personal assessment of our state of well being. Media images citing New Years Resolutions with great guarantees in part stimulate these concerns. For many of us, part of our assessment will include an annual or semi-annual physical exam which usually provides reassurance that everything is normal. Our doctors are happy with us. They can find no physical exam or laboratory abnormalities that provide cause for concern. Except for maybe our cholesterol level. But, we can easily explain this away by sheepishly admitting that we have not been careful with our food choices and promise to make more healthy food choices in the future.

Yet in the back of our mind, some of us know that the aging process is catching up with us. No one likes to admit to this feeling and so it remains in our subconscious. Many of us are so busy with our daily lives that we do not recognize it until mid-life. This unconscious fear is especially true for those of us who try to stay active and healthy. By mid-life this feeling is no longer subconscious, but common sense because everybody knows that aging is a natural progression of life. Either consciously or unconsciously, we correlate weight gain to a less youthful appearance. Surprisingly, This correlation is very predictive of our overall health and longevity.

As a matter of fact, many longevity experts believe that we now have the ability to extend our life span to well over one hundred years on average. This conclusion is largely due to the redirected effort by our medical community toward preventative health issues. Importantly, this does not mean that we will look older for a longer period of time, but rather that we will keep our youthful appearance longer. A very significant component of the secret to extend our life span is for us to keep our weight gain to a minimum.

The pure fact that there is a plethora of medical data about the lethal effects of being over weight has provided us with impetus to seek further understanding. For example, current evidence demonstrates that weight gain is now an independent risk factor for chronic and terminal diseases such as hypertension, heart attack, stroke, diabetes, and certain forms of cancer. This evidence has convinced many physicians to pay mor attention to their patients weight. How much we weigh is now considered to be as important a vital sign as our blood pressure.

For what ever reason, however, we the people of the United States of America seem to care less and less about how much we weigh. This statement may sound strong but it is backed by the documented fact that one out of every three of us is presently over weight. Whereas, only fifteen years ago one individual in four attained this lofty status. So, it turns out that our intuitive nature and unconscious fear is correct. Each time we tip the scale and see weight gain, our youthful appearance is indeed

3

slipping away.

Of course, weight gain is considered normal as we age, but only on the order of less than one pound a year after the age of twenty. Many of us know, however, that over the past two or three years we have gained at least ten or fifteen pounds. And for some of us, this can be particularly complexing, because we truly maintain a healthy diet and exercise program. For others well, there are countless reasons which may explain the weight gain. In order to effectively lose weight, we must first understand what causes weight gain.

For everyone of us the reason we gain more than a pound a year is multi-factorial, which means that more than one risk factor is involved. This Risk Factor Theory summarizes weight gain into five risk factors. These include Food Selection, Physical Activity, Stress, Metabolism, and Fat Utility.

Food Selection and Stress are refined terminology for caloric intake, while Physical Activity and Metabolism classically consist of our caloric expenditure. Fat Utility is not a reflection of either input nor output, but our genetic makeup. As you may know, the number one risk for becoming over weight is whether our parents are over weight or not. Importantly, each factor is not independent of one another, and certain interrelations between factors may escalate weight gain.

By recognizing that there is more than one factor to blame for weight gain, we are able to gain insight and control over two important aspects. First, it enables us to understand why many of our weight loss attempts are not successful. Second and most importantly, it enables us to make a systematic effort to minimize each category in order to maximize weight loss and extend our longevity. If you are experiencing weight gain of three or more pounds a year, then this step wise program should be seriously entertained.

Excitement is definitely in the air, and there are many reasons why so much optimism is present in the medical weight loss community. For one, we now understand weight loss theory at a detailed level. Importantly, we now have the ability to successfully treat the risk factors Food Selection, Metabolism, Stress, and Fat Utility. In addition, we know much more than ever before about Food Selection and Physical Activity, and how they correlate to weight loss and longevity.

However, most of us can achieve weight loss safely and painlessly without becoming an athletic track star or requiring constant medical supervision or procedures. Thus, our goal today is to get you started on a program that will improve your longevity and quality of life. To do this, we suggest that you begin The Cycle Diet and Program at your earliest convenience starting on Chapter 13. The remaining text will help you more fully understand which risk factors are inhibiting you from attaining your desired weight. Importantly, The Cycle Diet and Program can easily be incorporated into our daily life and will minimize each of the five risk factors that cause weight gain, maximizing your weight loss and extending your longevity.

Chapter 2

Caloric Restriction: When we decide to lose weight, one of the first things we will try to do is reduce the amount of calories we consume. This is translated into a positive effect on the risk factor Food Selection. Initially, most of us are able to participate for at least a week and find some success by noticing a few pounds have evaporated. In most cases, a reduction in calories will also reduce the amount of carbohydrates we consume. This in turn will allow fat cells to release fatty acids to be used to run our resting metabolism. However, our body detects that we are feeding it less, and consequently, our metabolism slows down in an effort to conserve energy. This is achieved by reducing the amount of the hormone, thyroxine, that is secreted by our thyroid gland. Our resting metabolism is only able t slow down by a few hundred calories per day. However, because our metabolism slows down, weight loss also slows down. Hence, caloric reduction has a negative effect on the risk factor Metabolism. In addition, internal stress may increase during caloric deprivation. We may notice that we are more irritable or grumpy. Anxiety and nervousness can also increase, which may increase our chance to binge eat. Thus, during episodes of caloric reduction, we tend to have a higher chance of resorting to binge eating. This is a normal behavior or response during these situations. The will power and or how we redirect stress during these situations may be different from person to person. Reducing the amount of calories we consume usually has a negative effect on the risk factor Stress.

The overall impact caloric restriction has on the five risk factors is to negatively affect Stress and Metabolism risk factors while Physical Activity and Fat Utility risk factors are not effected. Our goal to maximize successful weight loss is to positively affect these risk factors. The Five Risk Factor Theory shows us why most of us fail at a diet that is based entirely on caloric restriction.

Physical Activity: By increasing our activity, studies have shown that we will improve a large variety of health parameters such as improved quality of sleep reduction in anxiety, a decrease in nervousness, and improved self image. Consequently, every day stress that might precipitate eating when we are not hungry may not be signaled. Thus, physical activity has a positive effect on the risk factor Stress. If every time we get stressed out and felt the urge to eat something, but instead walked ten minutes or up and down stairs for two minutes, then we would put a big dent in weight gain. In all actuality, our inherent positive reward system which directs us to eat during times of stress, reduces stress for only a fraction of the time compared to physical activity.

Physical activity may, however, gradually increase the amount of calories we will desire to consume. Although, recent studies have shown that females usually increase their caloric intake and males will decrease their intake following exercise.

However, our resting metabolism will typically increase by at least 100 calories per day, which may signal us to desire more food. Remember, our body does not desire to lose weight, even when we exercise. The Fat Utilization Risk is not changed by an increase in activity.

The overall impact of increasing the Physical Activity Risk factor includes a positive weight loss affect on the Stress and Metabolism Risks as well, while negatively affecting only the Food Selection Risk factor. This is why we (as well as all clinical studies that have been completed) will clearly demonstrate weight loss just by increasing our activity even if the increased activity is minimal.

Combination of Caloric Restriction plus Exercise: The most recent combination study completed showed that a significant amount of weight can be lost during the first year, approximately 20 pounds on average. The overall impact during the first year can be summarized by the Food Selection and Physical Activity Risks receiving a positive effect while the risk factors Stress and Metabolism are neutralized. Fat Utilization is not effected.

However, the second year proved to be more difficult in that on average 15 pounds were regained. The reason for this is that caloric restriction is very difficult to maintain because internal stress will continually build, especially if less that 1300 calories are consumed daily. This unfortunately leads to increased episodes of binge eating as well as consuming when given any opportunity. Self control may be nonexistent during the second year. In these situations, food selection is also adversely effected, because we will tend to eat on impulse which leads to poor food selections such as carbohydrate and fat combination food groups. This type of food will temporarily reduce stress, because our body views it as a positive reward. However, carbohydrate and fat combination food groups are also detrimental because the produce the fastest weight gain. Due to our occasional indiscretions, we may become discouraged and eventually be less adherent to our caloric restrictive diet. This will double the negative impact on the Food Selection Risk because both the amount and type of food we consume will be adversely influenced.

During the second year, the Food Selection and Stress Risk factors slowly develop to adversely affect the weight loss program. Metabolism on the other hand has increased because the Food Selection Risk favors weight gain. Hence, the net result of this two year study of caloric reduction and exercise showed that weight loss was not successful past one year.

Perfect Program: Obviously the perfect program is one in which each of the five risk factors favor weight loss. This can clearly be achieved by a medical weight loss program or procedure. However, until now, there has not been a program available that can claim to positively effect all five risk factors long term without medical help. The weight loss achieved with The Cycle Diet and Program is designed to be a significant improvement over the caloric restriction and physical activity diet studies by improving the ability to keep the weight off. This can be achieved by cycling specific food groups. With The Cycle Diet, weight loss can safely achieve as much as 10 pounds a month with minimal effort.

Chapter 3

For at least one third of the US population the answer is yes to the question are you over weight. Many of us believe that how much we should weigh is not an exact science. Do we deny this subconsciously? This belief however, is far from the truth. Just like our blood pressure or cholesterol, how much we weigh also has normal limits. For whatever reason, obesity is not aggressively treated, unlike other chronic disease states. Over the past ten or so years, however, many of us have become more aware of the lethal effects being over weight can produce. The medical community is continually studying how much we weigh, and how this correlates with age and cause of death. In addition, most physicians understand how our weight relates to causes of morbidity such as diabetes, hypertension, heart disease, stroke, and cancer.

The most sensitive and standard way to determine if we are over weight is called Body Mass Index, BMI. This numerical value is generated from our height and weight. Table 1 below, will allow you to determine your BMI. Intersect your approximate height (shown in the left column, in feet and inches) with your approximate weight (shown in the top row, in pounds).

Table 1: Determining Your approximate BMI.

Weight	95	110	140	170	200	230	260	290	320
58"	20	23	29	35	41	47			
60"		21	27	33	39	45	51		
62"		19	25	31	37	43	49		
64"		18	24	29	34	40	45		
66"			22	27	32	37	42	47	
68"			21	26	30	35	40	45	
70"			20	25	29	33	37	41	
72"				23	27	31	35	39	43
74"				22	26	30	34	37	41
76"				21	25	28	32	35	39

If your approximate BMI is 26 or higher than you are considered over weight. It is as simple as that. If it is above 26 then you are at an increased risk for developing high blood pressure, diabetes, high cholesterol, heart disease, a heart attack, and certain forms of cancer. If your BMI is above 30, then clearly your weight is considered an independent risk factor for the above morbidity's and can definitely decrease your longevity. The evidence for this is decisive and is based on an extensive retrospective study of thirty years from a multi-center population.

In addition, our BMI and age can be related to our lowest risk of mortality. This information tells us our ideal range of weight in order for ours to minimize our health risks at any age, Table 2. Identify your approximate age by the top row (YR). The number under your age represents your optimal Body Mass Index (BMI). Surprisingly, both females and males follow this pattern for lowest overall

13

mortality rate. In general, females look most aesthetically pleasing at a BMI between 20 to 23, while males range from 25 to 27 to most people. We can use Table 1 to convert this BMI back into pounds by finding the closest BMI in our height row.

Table 2: Age, Body Mass Index, and lowest mortality.

YR	20	25	30	35	40	45	50	55	60	65	70
BMI	19	20	21	22	23	24	24.5	25	26	27	28

Another helpful tool to determine if we are over weight is percent body fat. The American College of Sports Medicine recommends the following body fat range for the age groups shown in the top row of Table 3.

Table 3: Recommended percent body fat based on age.

Age	20-29	30-39	40-49	50-59	60+
Females	16-24%	17-25%	19-28%	22-31%	22-33%
Males	7-17%	12-21%	14-23%	16-24%	17-25%

The combination of all three of the above measurements are the most accurate way we know to follow weight loss or weight gain. Percent body fat is especially useful once we have our BMI at or below 27. This is because it can accurately be used to shape our figure. During medical supervised weight loss, this measurement should be evaluated monthly. A determination can then be made to see if we are losing the right type of weight, i.e. fat pounds. Another more indirect way to determine if we are losing fat pounds is by monitoring how our clothes fit.

Write the numerical number that correlates to your Body Mass Index from Table 1, and optimal BMI for your age from Table 2 down in the space below. This will tell you how much weight you need to lose.

Chapter 4

Food Selection Risk factor applies to what type and amount of carbohydrate, protein and fat we consume. For over half of us, this risk factor is likely to be the single most important risk. The reason for its great impact on our weight is due to the fact that many external factors indirectly influence what we eat. Uncontrollable factors such as where we work, the type of work we do, where we live, how old we are, media and advertisements, beliefs about food, gender, race, economic status and s forth, indirectly shape our diet. In addition, the probability that we will change jobs because we are gaining weight, or turn the television off when something appetizing is displayed, are unlikely nor reasonable requests. They are important to understand, but considered beyond the scope of individual effort and should not deter you from trying to lose weight. Not withstanding the above, Food Selection is a very influential risk factor. As such, many of us can lose our desired weight just by following a few simple concepts about what we eat.

Food Selection is actually very interesting and is presented I some however brief, detail. It is defined to include the type and amount of energy intake (measured in calories). Energy intake is fundamentally categorized into three components which include Carbohydrates, Protein, and Fat. Thus, Food Selection literally applies to what type and amount of carbohydrate, protein, and fat we ingest. This truly is important, because there is mounting evidence which suggest that the type of food we select (not so much the caloric amount consumed daily) can significantly influence how much we weigh and our overall health and longevity.

The American Heart Association (AHA) recommends a diet consisting of roughly 55% carbohydrate, 15% protein, and less than 30% fat (10% saturated, 10% polyunsaturated, less than 15% mono-unsaturated). The recommended amount of daily energy intake is considered satisfactory between 1800 and 2200 calories. For most of us, these recommendations are reasonable in maintaining our weight. In addition, with this approximate caloric structure plus three and one half hours of moderate intensity activity a week, we can lose approximately one half of a pound per month for the first year. Continuing this program for a second year, we will succeed in keeping most of the weight we lost off, but not lose additional weight. For many of us, this recommendation is not very difficult to maintain. The rewards, nonetheless, are not that exciting nor motivation, especially if we need to lose thirty or forty pounds.

Further discomforting evidence suggest that a caloric reduction to less than 1300 calories per day will , on average, allow us to lose about a pound a month. Yet, for most of us this meager consumption is very difficult to maintain, and consequently, we will probably regain our weight back the following year.

17

To make weight loss even more difficult, we will desire to consume more calories each year for most of our life. The phenomenon is a primitive survival mechanism all humans share when there is an abundant food supply. For example, if you take a picture of your dinner plate with your normal serving size today, then compare it with a picture taken a year from now, you will probably notice that the latter picture contains larger portions. Even the people in France will surprisingly experience this observation.

Taking a moment to reflect on the above information. We can reasonably conclude that severe caloric restriction is futile because weight regain is inevitable, and an increase in activity, to what is recommended, may provide weight loss but only in the first year. As a matter of fact, the lower your percent body fat is, the more moderate-high physical activity you need to do daily. Medicinal enhancers typically allow us to achieve a low percent body fat with less moderate-high physical activity or shorter durations of moderate intensity activity.

When we examine these conclusions more closely with the five risk factors in mind, we can understand why caloric restriction by itself is almost always unsuccessful while even minimal activity can produce successful results, as outline in Chapter 2. It is also unlikely that severe caloric restriction plays a successful rule in unsupervised weight loss. However, conservative caloric restriction may be important towards this goal. Nevertheless, we will focus our discussion about the risk factor Food

Selection towards the type of carbohydrate, protein, or fat that we should ingest. This is because there is mounting evidence which suggest that the type of foods we select, not so much the amount we consume, can significantly influence how much we weigh and how long we live.

In summary, we believe that the key to increasing our longevity starts with weight loss. The Risk Factor Theory identifies five risk factors involved in weight gain. The Cycle Diet and Program enables us to make a systematic effort to maximize weight loss and improve longevity. The Risk Factor Theory helps explain the results of major scientific weight loss studies and the Cycle Diet was designed to improve the results of these studies and optimize our weight loss potential.

Chapter 5

The best way we have found to help you visualize how important carbohydrates are from a dietary perspective, is for you to imagine your body as a machine that runs by the least means of resistance. Therefore, if we need to expend energy, and have a choice between a carbohydrate, a protein, or a fat molecule then our body will choose the carbohydrate. This is because a carbohydrate requires less work for us to generate an energy molecule, namely Adenine Triphosphate or ATP. Simplistically, if carbohydrates are available then we will not use an alternate source of energy.

If we have a surplus of carbohydrates then our body will store them, and this storage is called glycogen. We, however, will continue to use some of the un-stored carbohydrates as energy to run our body, plus provide the energy to store a more potent energy source, namely fat. Importantly, the more glycogen we have stored, the more efficient our body becomes at storing fat. The reason for this is that fat contains at least twice the amount of energy that stored carbohydrate. This system is efficient. It makes sense from a survival perspective which is how our body views food, and is also why we continually store fat. The amount of carbohydrate we consume, therefore, plays an important role in fat storage and weight gain. Our available carbohydrate level (blood glucose level) is under the control of the hormone insulin. Hence, our blood insulin level ultimately decides what type of energy source we will use.

Conversely, as we deplete our glycogen storage, our body will more efficiently use stored fat as a source of energy and cause weight loss. During these instances, our blood insulin level is low. Therefore, we will want to conserve the remaining carbohydrates and thus, utilize more of our fatty acids stored in fat cells as the predominate source of expended energy. This concept is particularly important in weight loss theory, and our goal is to demonstrate how e can use this to our advantage.

Carbohydrates are, thus, the main fuel used. They are used either to expend energy (say provide the energy to walk to the store), or to store energy (in the form of glycogen and subsequently fat).

The AHA recommends approximately 1100 carbohydrate calories or 300 grams a day. In addition, The Food and Drug Administration (FDA) makes a distinguishment between the type of carbohydrate consumed. Their recommendations is for us to partake in more foods that are high in dietary and nondigestible fiber. Many grocery store items are required to document the dietary fiber, but not the nondigestible fiber content. Furthermore, a diet that is high in carbohydrates that do not have dietary fiber may be an independent risk factor for adult onset diabetes mellitus (AODM).

Fiber is typically associated with the carbohydrate group, except beans such as pinto, kidney and soy which are considered proteins. Most importantly, fibers have been shown to slow the carbohydrate absorption rate down, as well as decrease fat absorption. From a weight loss perspective, this is what we want. From a overall perspective of general health, carbohydrates that have fiber are important because the are also associated with various longevity markers such as improved bowel motility, a decrease in the incidence of colonic cancer, and improved cholesterol profile.

Carbohydrates are classified into two categories which are complex carbohydrates and simple carbohydrates. Complex carbohydrates or starches which include rice, potato, and pasta. Of these three, grained pasta and brown rice have higher levels of dietary fiber. Complex carbohydrates typically will also contain protein, minerals and vitamins. Simple carbohydrates which are defined here to be monosaccharides and sucrose (sugar cane) include soda pop, fruit drinks, fruit, and many nonfat candy, cookies, and pastries now available at the grocery store. Of these, fruit is likely to be the only one to have a significant amount of fiber, as well as protein, minerals and vitamins. They also have lower concentrations of simple carbohydrates, and are associated with antioxidants. Antioxidants are thought to decrease cellular damage and hence, increase cellular longevity. Blended fruit drinks, touted as health drinks, contain an enormous amount of simple carbohydrates.

The big problem with simple carbohydrates, from a dietary perspective, is that they will rapidly stop our body from using fat as an energy source. For example, when we are hungry, our body is efficiently using fat as a source of energy. Subsequently, by consuming any of the above simple carbohydrates, we will no longer utilize or burn fat. Candy, cookies, and pastries may or may not contain fat. The consumption of carbohydrate and fat combination products, in most situations, are not advantageous, because we are providing energy (the carbohydrate) to store fat.

In addition to the above foods, cereals, low fat crackers, and vegetables also consist predominantly of carbohydrates. They are however, a mixture of complex and simple carbohydrates (called combination carbohydrates) and have varying levels of fiber, protein, minerals and vitamins. Oat, wheat, and bran cereals, breads, and crackers, along with vegetables such as green beans, lettuce, carrots, celery, broccoli, and spinach can have significant levels of dietary and or nondigestible fibers. Recently, oat products have been found to be especially significant, because the dietary fiber they contain has been shown to impede saturated fat absorption and consequently lower our bad cholesterol (Low Density Lipoprotein or LDL).

Clearly, nondigestible fibers that are found in vegetables such as lettuce, carrots, cabbage, and celery are extremely beneficial. They increase bowel motility and can physically block fatty acids from getting absorbed through our gut lining. From a weight loss perspective, this is what we want. As mentioned, nondigestible fiber is typically not labeled

23

on food items.

Many vegetables are also associated with antioxidants, and from this perspective, any palatable vegetable may be beneficial to us. As mentioned, the reason we like antioxidants is because they decrease cellular damage, and increase cellular longevity. These phytochemicals which are found mainly in fruits and vegetables seem to decrease our risk for many types of cancers, as well as inhibit the free radical reactions involved in cardiovascular disease. For instance, lycopene which is found in tomatoes may decrease our risk for prostate cancer. The isothiocyanates found in turnips, watercress, and cabbage may hinder carcinogens. Flavanoids that are found in soy bean, bulb vegetables, and garlic are also considered anti-cancer and antiviral agents. The polyphenols in black tea and green tea and wine seem to disarm free radicals in arteries and the gastrointestinal tract which may lower the incidence of GI cancer and stroke. Spinach is loaded with beta carotene and vitamin E, which have also been shown to affect the incidence of certain forms of cancer and reduce cardiovascular disease in certain age groups. Vegetables loaded with folate can decrease the level of homocysteine which may reduce our risk for coronary artery disease. Recent evidence suggest, however, that some phytochemicals in vitamin supplement form may not have the same benefits, also see Appendix.

From a dietary perspective, there is no conclusive scientific data supporting the assumption that complex carbohydrates without dietary fiber, provide a benefit over monosaccharides or vice a versa. Complex carbohydrates clearly undergo some form of energy expenditure process by our digestive enzymes to produce simple carbohydrates so they can pass through our gut lining. The energy expended for this conversion is probably insignificant. However, complex carbohydrates typically contain more protein, minerals and vitamins than simple carbohydrates. As mentioned previously, over consumption of complex carbohydrates without fiber may precipitate diabetes. Complex carbohydrates without dietary fiber surge thru the digestive lining and is not considered helpful during weight loss.

Simple carbohydrates, mostly in the form of glucose, are what our body requires to generate energy, ATP. This carbohydrate form is readily absorbed through our digestive lining and into the blood stream, and is why a hypoglycemic patient finds rapid symptomatic relief by ingesting orange juice or sucking on hard candy. The rate of glucose absorption is delayed for complex carbohydrates which is why we do not typically give pasta or rice to these patients. After absorption, glucose then passes to the liver where it has three fates. It can be converted to glycogen or stored glucose, or can help produce triglycerides to be stored in fat cells and cause weight gain, or it can remain in the blood stream as glucose to be used by peripheral tissue as energy, ATP. what our liver does with glucose depends on what we need at any given time.

The hormone insulin, in essence, tells glucose where it is needed. This hormone therefore controls our metabolic state, which should not be confused with metabolism. Recognizing that our metabolic state is constantly changing is important. For example, our metabolic state when we are hungry will be different than when we are not hungry. The sensation of hunger usually correlates with a low blood glucose and insulin level. A low insulin level will send a message to our brain telling us that we need to eat something. This is because our body is using more fat than desired. So, our metabolic state during times of hunger is typically when we are using the most fat as a source of energy. Hence, our insulin level controls what type of energy we will use. When it is low we will use fat but when it is high we will use carbohydrate.

In summary, our body loves to run on carbohydrates. Storage levels of carbohydrates called glycogen, play a very significant role in what the liver does with it. As this level nears capacity, we are able to store fat very efficiently. Conversely, as the glycogen level nears depletion, our body is able to use fat most efficiently, as energy. Therefore, the amount of carbohydrate we consume can strongly influence weight loss, maintenance, or weight gain. Importantly our body will not use fat as energy unless it perceives that our carbohydrate level is low. This system is ultimately regulated by our blood insulin level and receptors thereof. In addition, we will promptly shut off fat breakdown or lipid lysis when simple carbohydrates are consumed. Carbohydrates associated with fibers are favorable, because they slow the rate of glucose absorption down and decrease the amount of fat that can be absorbed. Examples include brown rice, grained pasta, most vegetables, salads, as well as low fat cereals, crackers, and breads that contain oat, wheat, or bran.

Chapter 6

Most of the dietary protein we consume is not used by our body as an energy source. Its predominant function is to provide building blocks for processes like but not limited to, protein synthesis for enzyme replacement, replacement of damaged cells in blood and shedding organs like skin and intestinal mucosa, as well as intestinal secretions. Surprisingly, very little protein is required for muscle growth and maintenance. In addition, our body reuses the components of proteins called amino acids, and collectively they are termed the protein turnover pool. Consequently, we do not require an extraordinary amount of protein to survive. The reason why our body utilizes protein so efficiently is because it is the most important ingredient we consume, from a survival perspective. We need the machine before we can put gas in it.

Our body can, however, use protein as a source of energy. Importantly, protein has the capability to be transformed into glucose or a glucose intermediate, whereas fat cannot. This is surprisingly important because some of our vital organ systems prefer glucose as a way to generate energy. However, it is different than carbohydrate or fat in that, we do not store protein for the sole purpose of generating available energy or ATP.

A diet that is high in protein, for example, but also contains available carbohydrates and fats can still produce unwanted fat pounds. This is because our body will use the excess protein as available energy to store more fat. As mentioned, our body is very efficient with protein, and will not want to waste it. Since it is not stored like glycogen or fat, our extra protein we consume is turned into energy or ATP.

On the other hand, when our carbohydrate storage or glycogen level is low, much like the initial stages of caloric restriction or starvation, we will first use the carbon structures of protein to generate glucose intermediates or glucose and subsequently produce ATP. Initially, the amount of fat used will not be affected much. In essence, protein components from the protein turnover pool are used to help out the carbohydrates with satisfying our energetic needs. This process changes our metabolic state to breakdown mode or catabolic state and is very similar to the way carbohydrates generate ATP in that protein will use common pathways. Protein is obviously not as efficient as the carbohydrate in generating ATP. In other words, we consume more energy converting protein into ATP than we do with glucose into ATP.

In simplistic terms, a protein will take two steps to get to the energy source of ATP, while carbohydrates take only one step to ATP. Remember, our body runs on the least means of resistance, and hence prefers the one step process. From a dietary perspective, we prefer to use the two step process because it uses more energy. Thus, protein consumption can indirectly increase our resting metabolic rate and help minimize the risk factor

Metabolism.

During the initial stages of caloric deprivation, we will only use protein as the predominant energy producer preferential to fat for a limited time, approximately twelve hours. This is because protein has limited storage and a higher level or survival responsibility associated with its function when compared to fat. In fact, the proteins being utilized during the initial stages of caloric reduction come from our daily protein turnover pool. Remember, we normally do not store protein, and under optimal conditions it is not required to produce energy.

Past twelve or so hours, our carbohydrate storage will be depleted. Fatty acids released from fat cells will now be the predominant type of energy used to run our resting metabolic rate. However, we will continue to use protein to generate glucose, but at a slower rate. This is because some of our organ systems prefer glucose as it source of energy, like our brain, adrenal gland, and red blood cells. Remember, protein can make glucose, where as fat cannot make glucose. When we are using fat as a source of energy, our body will also use protein. Thus, as long as we continue to consume protein products, we will always maintain a turnover pool of protein. This concept is important to understand during weight loss, especially if we want to avoid gastrointestinal problems. In addition, we do not want our body to perceive that the protein turnover pool is low or depleted.

Our body, however, will rapidly stop using protein and fat if we consume a moderate amount of carbohydrates. This represents a switch back to the metabolic state we are most comfortable with. Consequently, we will again begin to use carbohydrates to store fat. There is no way for us to burn fat if carbohydrates are in our system at an appreciable level.

Dietary intake of protein predominantly comes from meat, which includes beef in select and choice cuts, pork and ham, chicken, turkey, seafood, and fish. Beans such as soy, pinto, and kidney are also classified in this category. Certain dairy products such as one percent or non fat milk and cheese, eggs, and low fat low carbohydrate yogurt are also proteins.

The total amount of protein recommended by the AHA is around 80 grams or 300 calories a day, which is more than what we require under normal circumstances. The FDA recommends that we consume more proteins that are associated with fiber. A diet lacking in protein, but sufficient in carbohydrates and fat is called Kwashiorkor. Physical manifestations of this syndrome includes retention of fat, edema, moon shaped face, poor hair color and texture, and dry skin. It may also be associated with personality changes such as irritability and apparent lack of feelings or expression.

Compared to other meats, white fillet fish, turkey and chicken breast are associated with the lowest content of fat and vary from no fat to five or six percent. However, over the past ten or so years, beef has significantly reduced its percent of fat. Select cuts which include eye of round, round tip toploin, tenderloin, and sirloin all contain around four percent fat. Choice and prime cuts are approximately seven and eleven percent respectively Hence, when comparing the fat content of meats, beef has become surprisingly competitive, with the exception of hamburger. Clearly, the amount of beef and pork we consume should reflect our personal cholesterol profile. Ham is typically low in fat, but may contain high levels of unwanted sodium. Chicken and turkey have the lower levels of saturated fat compare to beef and pork, while shrimp is loaded with polyunsaturated fat.

Brown beans such as pinto and kidney, and soy or tofu provide a high source of protein with generally low quantities of fat. They also contain low to moderate quantities of carbohydrates and dietary fiber. Low and non fat dairy products are an excellent source of protein, but lack fiber. Eggs are actually lower in saturated fat than we previously believed, nonetheless, they contain high levels of cholesterol. Recent evidence suggests that saturated fatty acids elevate our LDL level at least five fold higher than does cholesterol.

When comparing the composition of protein products, we find that plant proteins found in beans and other vegetable products do not contain all the amino acids or building blocks for proteins that is required for normal cellular replacement and body rejuvenation. Physical signs of deficient amino acids that can only be acquired by dairy or animal protein consumption i.e. essential amino acids may become apparent in tissues and organs that undergo continual growth or shedding such as hair, nails, skin, and digestive linings. Thus, essential amino acids supplements should be considered when predominantly obtaining protein from plants. Notwithstanding, the combination of plant proteins plus dairy products will typically provide all the amino acids required for normal protein function.

Interestingly, males who consume more protein have been shown to have higher levels of testosterone than individuals who consume less quantities. Testosterone is significant in that it provides an a additional mechanism to utilize fat as a source of energy in protein synthesis and muscle growth. In addition, low blood levels of total testosterone is associated with increased abdominal fat and a HGH cholesterol profile. Furthermore, evidence suggests that by the age of 40, a significant number of males may have low or low normal testosterone levels.

Lastly, dietary protein contains a lot of nitrogen. Each amino acid contains at least one nitrogen atom, and hundreds of amino acids typically make up proteins. In excess, nitrogen is not good for our brain. For example, and individual who is on a high protein and low carbohydrate diet for an extended period may experience altered mental status if adequate water consumption is ignored. For an individual who has liver or kidney disease, or is taking prescription medication, should consult their primary care physician before engaging in a diet that lacks carbohydrates.

In summary, proteins is not a desired choice as an energy source. However, it may be used as an energy source, because it can be converted to glucose and subsequently used as energy when our glycogen or carbohydrate storage is low. For instance, when we are dieting by caloric restriction, our body is using protein as a source of energy in addition to fat. This is because some of our organs require glucose to generate energy. Thus, proper amounts of protein intake is important when dieting. Conversely, if carbohydrates are available then we will not use protein or fat to make energy. Dietary meats such as white fillet fish, chicken and turkey breast, as well as select and choice cuts of beef are a valuable source of protein. Plant proteins such as pint, kidney and soy beans are an excellent alternative and also contain fiber, but must be supplemented with vitamins containing essential amino acids or dairy products. Low and non fat dairy products without added carbohydrates are also beneficial.

Chapter 7

Our body perceives the accumulation of fat and consequential weight gain as its ultimate survival weapon against prolonged starvation. When we have adequate carbohydrates, we will stop storing them and begin to store fatty acids into fat cells at an increased rate. This is because there is at least two times the energy that can be reproduced from stored fat than from glycogen. For example, if our glycogen level is half full or fifty percent, then we may store only forty percent of digested fat. However, if our glycogen level is near capacity of eighty five percent , then we can store over eighty percent of it. So now we can understand why the amount of glycogen we have stored determines whether or not we will use fat as energy. This carbohydrate-fat relationship is a biochemical law that makes sense to our body because it is only concerned with staying alive. Therefore, if we have a diet that is high in carbohydrates and relatively low in fatty acids ten most , if not all, of the fatty acids we digest will go directly into our fat cells.

Classically, fatty acids are thought to continually be stored and released from fat cells all the time. Most of us store more than we release which typically results in an increase in fat pounds yearly. Since fat storage is important from a survival perspective, we do not release stored fat unless it is absolutely necessary. Clearly, if we were to consume little or no carbohydrates then our body would have no alternative but to release fatty acids. Carbohydrate deprivation is not good for us past two or three days.

Fat cells release fatty acids which are then utilized by other tissues to generate energy. As mentioned, fatty acids use a different biochemical pathway for them to generate energy than do carbohydrates or proteins. This pathway is termed beta oxidation, but not all organs are equipped to use this pathway. However, vital organs like our heart, kidneys, lungs, and muscle tissue rely on this pathway when our carbohydrate storage is perceived to be low. Fatty acids will also provide the energy required to convert protein into glucose so that glucose can be used to feed our brain and red blood cells.

Dietary fat is ingested in the form of glycerides, called saturated or unsaturated fatty acids. They are then bound together in groups of three to form triglycerides which are then ready to be stored in fat cells. Presently, the AHA recommends a diet consisting of less than thirty percent of fat from daily caloric intake, or approximately 600 calories or 75 grams. In general, saturated fats are what we try to avoid because of the associated risk with heart disease or plaque buildup in our arteries. Trans fatty acids are considered to be the most lethal, but many fatty foods do not contain large quantities. Hence, no more than 200 calories or 25 grams of the saturated ones should be consumed daily. The FDA has helped consumers identify food products that are high in saturated fats by making producers label them with their saturated and unsaturated content. From a dietary perspective, the release of saturated fats from fat cells require more energy than unsaturated fats. Therefore, saturated fats are less preferred, and more difficult to remove once incorporated into fat cells.

Rarely do we consume fat as an isolated product. Dietary fat predominately comes from meats, dairy products, cooking oil and margarine products, nuts , chips, chocolate, cookies, pastries, most candy and fast food products. Meat products such as hamburger and pork have a higher fat content, approximately twenty five percent, than the meats classified as proteins. Dairy products such as whole or two percent milk, ice cream, whipped cream, butter, most types of cheese, cookies, pastries, and candy are loaded with fat and ay also contain significant levels of sugar or simple carbohydrates. Remember, carbohydrate and fat combination products are the fastest way for us to gain fat ponds. Cooking oils and margarine consist solely of fat, and are not typically consumed by themselves. Chip products like potato and corn, as a rule contain abut one gram of fat per chip, and are also high in carbohydrates. In addition, they may contain high levels of sodium which make it difficult for us to eat just one. Nuts are also enormously high in fatty acids, but are polyunsaturated. Polyunsaturated fats are believed to play a protective role in heart disease. In addition, peanuts contain phenolic substances similar to green tea, black tea, and red wine. Fast food consumption has become an epidemic in America, and these products are typically loaded with saturated and trans fatty acids. It is not unusual for an

37

individual to consume over one thousand calories at a fast food restaurant , and still be hungry. Foods that are high in trans fatty acids include margarine, hydrogenated vegetable oil typically used in the preparation of cookies, snacks, chips, and french fries. Trans fatty acids are also associated with an increase risk of breast cancer.

Great strides over the last ten years, however, have been made in most of the above good groups to decrease the fat content in them. As mentioned, beef has reduced its fat content dramatically, select cuts are four percent fat, choice cuts are seven percent and prime cuts are about eleven percent. Dairy products have diversified to include low and non fat cheese, milk, yogurt, and ice cream. Cooking oils and margarine-like spread products are still high in fat, but are now predominately made from canola and soybean oil. Baked chips are now on the market, transferring them to the carbohydrate group. And recently, a different way to make chip products was marketed that minimized the fat absorption thru the gut but received minimal success because of the side effects.

As a matter of fact, Americans in general , have unconsciously decreased their fat intake by seven percent from 1975 to 1990 to a 33 percent daily intake. What is alarming, however, is that obesity has risen within the same time period by approximately 31 percent and now has become an even greater medical issue.

There is evidence that he amount of physical activity we do has decreased over the past twenty years. Approximately 800 calories a week due to walking has been cut out of our daily routine. One reason for this is that our employment has become increasingly more sedentary. Our urban lifestyle, has in some ways also decreased our ability and desire to do leisure physical activity. But intuitively, there has to be more to the story because this would mean that we have stopped moving all together. In addition, from what we have recently learned about the health benefits of moderate intensity activity, for most of us it is very difficult to avoid half of what is recommended just by getting up and going to work five days a week.

The fact that there is an enormous amount of food products available that are fat free may also be a contributing factor in the increase weight Americans are experiencing. Fat free products are usually high in carbohydrates which will make carbohydrate storage go up. As carbohydrate storage goes up, we are more efficient in storing fat. Thus, even though we have cut down our fat consumption significantly, by turning to carbohydrates as a substitute, we have effectively made our body more efficient in storing fat.

In summary, the amount of carbohydrates we consume determines how efficiently we will store fat. As our carbohydrate storage or glycogen level nears capacity, than fat storage increases its efficiency. Dietary intake of fats come from meats like hamburger and pork, dairy products, cooking oil and spreads, nuts, cakes,. pastries, chips, chocolate, and fast food. Saturated and trans fatty acids are a major health risk because of their strong association with heart disease and cancer. Fat content has been dramatically reduced over the past ten or more years in most of the above foods. Consequently, over the same time frame, fat consumption has decreased significantly. Seemingly paradoxical, however, is the fact that more people are considered over weight than ever before. One explanation is that we are more efficient at storing fat because we continue to substitute carbohydrate calories for fat calories.

Chapter 8

Over the past ten or so years, our lack of physical activity has taken most of the blame for the rapid trend in weight gain that our country is experiencing. Each of us tend to agree with this hypothesis because this belief is based on our own personal experience. For example, when a friend tells you that you look out-of-shape, the first thing that pops in your head of a constructive nature is the desire to start exercising. You may reminisce back to the time when you had your best physique, and also what your physical activity included. The problem with this hypothesis is that , the amount of physical activity required to get-in-shape is not likely to be the same amount needed for us to lose weight. In other words, our goal is not to turn you into an athlete like you once was, but to minimize or neutralize the Physical Activity Risk Factor.

Conversely for some of us, the weight will not disappear, no matter how much exercise we do. In these situations, our weight loss capabilities from physical activity is probably maximized, and other risk factors should be more fully addressed. Again, the goal is to not let this risk factor adversely affect our chances to lose weight. For many of us, the risk factor Physical Activity is surprisingly not the major impetus causing our weight gain. For example, just by jumping out of bed, getting ready for work, going to work, and coming home, we can fulfill at least half of the amount of physical activity recommended by the experts.

These experts have concluded that we only need two and one half to three and one half hours of moderate activity or one and one half hours of moderate to high activity a week in order to effectively neutralize the Physical Activity Risk Factor. An interesting conference was completed by The National Institute of Health (NIH) concerning physical activity and its relationship to our health and longevity. The experts involved in establishing our activity recommendations included specialists in cardiology, psychology, epidemiology, exercise physiology, geriatrics, nutrition, pediatrics, public health and sports medicine. They recommend that all children and adults should set a long term goal to accumulate at least thirty minutes or more of moderate intensity activity on most, or preferably all, days of the week. To most of us, this sounds like a lot of exercise, but actually it is not. This is because there are a lot of activities that we normally do on a daily basis which can qualify as moderate intensity activity.

Thirty minutes of moderate activity a day progressively improves longevity risks such as smoking, high blood pressure, high cholesterol, obesity, and diabetes. This means that if you smoke, your risk of dying from lung cancer is lowered by maintaining thirty minutes of activity a day. It can also lower your chances of gaining weight, and improve your blood pressure and cholesterol profile.

The fact that this activity can reduce weight gain

42

is an understatement. More recent evidence shows that on average, we can lose about seven pounds a year when we maintain two and one half hours of moderate activity a week. The success of this can be easily understood by relating it to our Five Risk Factors. This activity improves our resting metabolism by expending approximately one hundred extra calories a day. In addition, internal stress such as anxiety, nervousness, and personal self esteem are improved. Therefore, three risk factors are effected in a positive way, from the perspective of weight loss as outlined in Chapter 2.

What is really so significant, is that the majority of the health benefits of physical activity is gained by performing moderate activity. In addition, three separate ten minute bouts of activity is equivalent to thirty minutes. This concept is important to us because it provides us with the opportunity to incorporate quick activities into our busy schedules. You can even pretend that you are running behind schedule all day and there by picking up the pace..

Moderate activity is determined as being at least three calories expended per minute of activity. Intermittent or short bouts of five or ten minutes can include the normal tasks of daily living such as vacuuming, sweeping and mopping, cleaning windows and counter tops, child care, cleaning the garage, and washing the car. Most importantly, the walk required for us in going to and from work can count. We sometimes fail to appreciate that walking is moderate exercise and will consequently under estimate the amount we actually do. Taking the stairs instead of the elevator is extremely valuable, because the caloric expenditure is equivalent to jogging. Other more classical forms of moderate intensity activity include bike riding, swimming, roller skating or roller blading, tennis, golf, home repair, and gardening.

Moderate to high activities or having at least seven calories expended per minute include jogging, basketball, and soccer while high intensity activities like running which expends at least fifteen calories per minute are associated with an increased risk of injury, discontinuation of activity, or acute cardiac events during the activity. Clearly, the most active individuals have lower cardiovascular morbidity and mortality rates than do those who are least active. However, most of the benefit appears to be accounted for when comparing the least active individuals to those who are moderately active. This is particularly appealing to those of us who do not desire, nor have the time to spend endless hours in a gym. More importantly, by maintaining the amount of activity required by the NIH, we know that we have minimized this Risk Factor as it relates to weight gain. Those of us who have progressed, and now typically participate in moderate to high intensity activity, thirty minutes can be performed approximately three times weekly to achieve similar cardiovascular benefits.

Those of us who are currently sedentary or have minimal activity should gradually build up to the recommended goal of thirty minutes of moderate activity daily. For example, this can be done by adding a few minutes to our walk each day or gradually picking up the pace. We can also park our car a little further away from where we work or shop. This will reduce the risks associated with suddenly increasing the amount or intensity of exercise. Initiating a program that develops muscular strength and joint flexibility is also important, and improves our ability to perform tasks thus reducing the probability of injury. Upper extremity resistance or strength training can improve muscular function, balance, coordination, and agility, as well as provide cardiovascular benefits. Remember, the muscular-skeletal systems oxygen requirements is improved by both of these activities which translates to an increase in resting metabolic rate.

Increased physical activity appears to also benefit individuals with a prior heart attack, angina pectoris, peripheral vascular disease and congestive heart failure. Individuals who are currently sedentary, minimally active or presently taking prescription medication should consult their primary care physician for advise before starting a physical activity program.

In summary, we have the preconception that the lack of physical activity is the main cause of our weight gain. Thirty minutes of moderate intensity activity a day is considered sufficient to minimize our weight gain from what would normally be contributed by this Risk Factor. In addition, moderate activity will progressively minimize other longevity risks such as smoking, high blood pressure, high cholesterol, cardiovascular disease, and diabetes to name only a few. Examples of this type of activity include, vacuuming, child care washing your car, and walking. Importantly, we can do ten minute bouts of activity and this will count toward the two and one half to three and one half hours needed weekly. This also provides us with the opportunity to incorporate quick activities into our busy schedule. Short bouts of upper extremity resistance training is equivalent to moderate intensity activity.

Chapter 9

One of the more fascinating aspects of weight loss theory is how we are drawn to food as a response to perceived stress. Stressful situations compel us to behave differently than we normally would given a less stressful situation. When we experience stress, each of us will try various different ways to respond or deal with it. Our behavior may produce a positive or negative reward or outcome. What we perceive as good or bad is largely related to social and public laws, however, it may also be dependent on each individual.

A negative reward will typically decrease the chance that we will respond the same if a similar situation arises. For example, social awareness and public laws have decreased the occurrence of Americans driving motor vehicles under the influence of alcohol. On the other hand, if we respond to a particular stimuli and that response leads to a positive reward then there is an increased chance that we will respond similarly given the same stimulus. This means that, throughout our lifetime, we will unconsciously search out positive reward systems in response to stress. Furthermore, we may expand this response to cover different stimuli so to achieve the same reward.

For most of us our body has a sophisticated inherent positive reward system built-in that directs us to eat when placed in situations which we consciously or unconsciously perceive to be stressful. Hence, this positive reinforcement may result in an increase frequency of eating, and unknowingly we may become addicted to its rewards. Thus stress can have a considerable impact on how much we weigh. Simplistically, our body wants us to feed it, and from a survival perspective this mechanism provides assurance that we will consume food. Therefore, our reward system likely exists so that we will unconsciously desire food. So, even if we forget to eat, this system will eventually remind us. However, there are a few individuals which is a subgroup of Anorexia Nervosa whom may not have their positive reward system functioning properly. Consequently, they do not receive gratification from food consumption and hence may eventually starve themselves to death.

From a dietary perspective, daily stress is defined to include any environmental or internal stimuli which leads to an increased frequency of eating whether the act is conscious or not. We normally do not equate boredom, for example, with stress. However, this situation increases our chance of eating when we are not hungry. Therefore, it is defined under the Stress Risk Factor. For many of us, there are numerous response to cover different stimuli. In other situations, however, stress may trigger appetite suppression or a decreased frequency of food consumption. How stress affects you may be different than how it affects your friend or family member. Thus, not everybody responds the same to a given situation or stimulus, and there are an infinite number of stimuli which generate a response. Therefore, this risk factor continues to be studied. Yet, we understand some environmental and internal stimuli which lead to an increased frequency of eating. In addition, we more fully understand the positive reward system our body uses to make us desire food.

Environmental stimuli that may cause us to eat more frequently include boredom, busy schedule, social situations, entertainment activities such as watching televison, and the amount of time we spend near the kitchen. This is typically the stimuli that causes food consumption when we are not hungry. Such situations can be particularly troublesome to those of us who have difficulty keeping weight off because they may trigger an internal stimulus. For example, you may feel uncomfortable around a group of acquaintances which direct you to respond by eating a few to many appetizers. This in turn may trigger anxiety or guilt. We feel anxious or guilty because we know that it will cause weight gain. The fact that anxiety can be relieved temporarily by food tells your body that you are receiving a positive reward, and hence may lead to further food consumption. Paradoxically, we are quickly reminded that this behavior will result in weight gain, which is aesthetically unpleasant and anxiety may increase. The cyclic nature of this internal conflict resembles a mild form of an obsessive compulsive disorder called a Binge Disorder. Normally, every one of us will binge eat from time to time. However, this disorder may be difficult to overcome, depending on the severity.

Internal stimuli that may result in an increase in food consumption include anxiety, cravings, nervousness, personal self esteem, and mood or mental state of mind. Clearly, an argument can be made that environmental stimuli should be included with internal stimuli. This is because an environmental stimulus may trigger an internal stimulus which in turn generates a response. Hence, they commonly work together. However, our recognition that certain environmental stimuli, without an internal stimuli, can be easily fixed by avoiding that situation. We may not, however, have similar control over the internal stimuli that we feel daily, regardless of the situation. Therefore, even if we recognize the internal stimulus that is causing an increased frequency of eating and understand the conflict that we are experiencing, we may feel helpless about its effect. Fortunately, we understand many of the biochemical mechanisms that illicit internal stimuli. In addition, since many environmental stimuli trigger a specific internal stimulus and then produce a response or behavior, then we only need to treat the internal stimulus to deter the response. As mentioned, some environmental stimuli will directly produce a response and therefore behavior modification can be successful in these situations.

Many foods produce drug-like effects on our body. Some have the ability to alter an individuals mood and or affect pleasure centers located in the brain. To some extent, this is one way we are compelled to consume food. For example, spicy food and chocolate are thought to elevate levels of endorphins which may illicit a mild euphoric state. High doses of simple carbohydrates in combination with fat may also follow this mechanism. Pastries, candy bars, cookies and dairy products like ice cream are all examples that illicit a similar state. We may perceive this feeling as pleasurable and thus consider their consumption as a positive reward. In addition, the consumption of such products may further produce an overwhelming desire to re-illicit that feeling. Hence, we may find ourselves craving certain foods. An extreme example of this would be a heroin user that is experiencing withdrawal symptoms, and finds temporary relief from craving by consuming large doses of pastry products. Although we are unlikely to relate to this example, it does point out just how strong these drug-like foods have on internal stimuli.

In addition, complex carbohydrates or high doses of simple carbohydrates are believed to indirectly elevate levels of the neurotransmitter, serotonin. Serotonin produces an overall calming and sometimes sedating effect on you. This sensation is extremely important in our sophisticated inherent positive reward system, because it provides relief from internal stimuli such as nervousness and anxiety. It is , nonetheless, problematic because the effect is only temporary or transient. In addition to the calming effect elevated Serotonin levels produce, it can also relieve cravings and trigger a fullness sensation which may be gratifying. Complex carbohydrates without dietary fiber such as potatoes, pasta and white rice are well known to produce a sedative effect. Furthermore, by adding a cream sauce to them, we may generate an additional euphoric feeling. Especially addicting, are the complex carbohydrate and fat combinations that have moderate levels of salt added to them, such as chip products, some crackers, french fries, and pizza. From a dietary perspective, carbohydrates and fat combination foods are the fastest way our body knows how to add fat pounds. However, our body does not view this as a problem because it does not desire to lose weight. It is very important for us to realize that our body knows that it will live longer with more fat pounds should we for any reason decide to stop eating.

Less is known about what drives us to eat protein products and how it relates to our inherent positive reward system. Clearly, our body should have some desire mechanism in place because protein is considered the most important caloric ingredient needed for proper daily function. Although, as mentioned previously, under normal circumstances our body does not require large amounts of protein on a daily basis. This is because we reuse amino acids, or building blocks or protein. There is some speculation that protein consumption may cause a transient elevation of the essential amino acid, Tyrosine, which may elevate levels of the neurotransmitters norepinephrine and dopamine. The affect of this elevation is not typically considered addicting. For example, elevated levels of norepinephrine results during fight or flight situations, such as when we are confronted by a stranger unexpectedly. Intuitively, we do not like this feeling and probable try to avoid this stimuli.

In summary, The Stress Risk Factor may cause an increased frequency of eating, especially when we are not hungry. The reason for this is because our body has a sophisticated inherent positive reward system which can transiently relieve daily stress after we consume certain foods. Environmental stimuli such as, boredom, social situations, and entertainment activities can generally be minimized by behavior modification. Internal stimuli such as nervousness, anxiety, and cravings are more difficult to change through behavioral restructuring. Certain foods may produce a mild euphoric sensation by triggering endorphin-like pathways. We perceive this as pleasurable, giving these products an addicting quality to their consumption. They may include chocolate, pastries, and candy bars, as well as other items that have high doses of simple carbohydrates such as potato, pasta, and high concentrations of simple carbohydrates can indirectly elevate serotonin levels. This neurotransmitter is extremely important in our inherent reward system because it produces a calming almost sedating feeling as well as a fullness sensation which may be gratifying. Thus, we may unconsciously attempt to self medicate ourselves with carbohydrates, which elevate serotonin levels in order to feel better. Unfortunately, carbohydrate and fat combination foods, when consumed frequently, can cause rapid weight gain.

Chapter 10

While you are sitting on the couch and reading this book, you are expending energy. We define this as our resting metabolic rate. During respiration, we consume oxygen, which in turn is used to help generate energy (Adenosine Triphosphate, ATP) to run our bodily functions. The expended energy also produces heat, and is a reflection of our body core temperature. Metabolic rate can also be grossly measured by other external physical signs such as respiration and heart rate. Importantly, no one has the same resting metabolic rate. Even if there exists a small difference between individuals, the rate of energy expenditure can add up over time. For example, individual A has a resting metabolic rate of 1900 calories per day while individual B expends 1925 calories. In a month, individual B has expended approximately 750 more calories than individual A. Hence, if all other risk factors are equal and an initial BMI that is equal between individual's A and B, we would expect individual A to eventually weigh more than individual B.

Our hormones are to blame for the variation we observe when comparing resting metabolic rates. The two most important hormones that influence our metabolism are insulin and thyroxine. Insulin is secreted by the pancreas when our body perceives that the glucose level in the blood has increased. The net effect of this from a dietary perspective is to store fat.

Conversely, and under normal functioning situations, our blood insulin level is low when the blood glucose level is low. This metabolic state signals fatty acid release from fat cells and protein conversion to glucose or an intermediate of glucose to be used as energy. We therefore have some control over insulin's effect on our metabolism by what type of food we consume.

We have less control over the effects of thyroxine. Thyroxine is secreted by our thyroid, and is the major factor that influences the metabolic rate of all our tissues. Comparatively, the amount secreted daily is different in each individual. Yet, your thyroxine level is likely to be considered within normal limits if you go to your primary care physician to get it checked. For females, recent evidence suggests that a baseline Thyroid Stimulating Hormone (TSH) level drawn at the age of thirty.

Increased levels of thyroxine cause fatty acid release from fat cells, glycogen conversion to blood glucose and protein conversion to glucose or glucose intermediates. All of which is used to produce ATP or energy to be expended. Consequently, acutely elevated levels of this hormone raise our core body temperature , and also increase our heart rate and force of contraction of the heart, as well as increase respiration rate. Chronically elevated levels above normal limits are typically not considered beneficial to the longevity of our heart, and is the main reason why the use of thyroxine for weight loss is considered unsatisfactory. High-normal levels also increase the sensitivity to the neurotransmitters epinephrine and norepinephrine and this combination with thyroxine is believed to provide an amplified effect compared to the collective separate effect. Decreased levels of thyroxine is seen during caloric restriction which makes sense since your metabolic rate will decrease to conserve energy. Decreased levels is also seen during the use of oral glucocorticoids like prednisone, and hypertensive medication such as beta blockers.

To understand our metabolism a little better, we need to know how much energy each organ system consumes at resting state. We can divide our organ systems up to include our skeletal muscle, abdominal organs, heart, kidneys, brain and skin. The two organs that consume the most energy at rest are our skeletal muscle and abdominal organs which equal approximately sixty to seventy percent, depending on our muscle mass. The remainder is predominantly shared between our heart, kidneys, brain, and skin. Interestingly, the energy required for our brain is surprisingly constant no matter what activity we are doing. We can be either in deep thought or day dreaming and expend the same amount of energy.

Our metabolism is also dependent on our daily activities. The amount of energy used by our body at a resting state is obviously less than what is required to complete a task such as walking to the near by store. Thus, our resting metabolic rate plus the energy consumed to complete our daily activities is equal to the total amount of energy expended that day. Importantly, the resting energy required for the average person generally consists of approximately eighty to eighty-five percent of the total energy expended per day. This is not true for elite athletes or individuals who spend more than two hours of moderate-high intensity activity daily.

When we participate in some type of physical activity, the two organ systems that are largely affected is our skeletal muscle and heart. They increase their energy requirements, while our abdominal organs, kidneys, brain, and skin stay relatively constant. As a matter of fact, during resistance exercise and or moderate intensity activity, our skeletal muscle requires more than five times the amount of energy than during our resting state. Hence, the amount of energy required just to satisfy our skeletal muscle needs is greater than two times the total amount of our overall resting metabolic rate. What is even more significant is that ten to fifteen hours after completion of this activity, our resting metabolic rate is on average, five to seven percent higher that normal. This translates to at least one hundred extra calories expended per day. Moderate-high intensity activity when performed on a regular basis can effectively maximize our metabolic rate, and thus, remove this risk factor, as well as the Physical Activity risk factor from the weight gain equation. Conversely, the more sedentary we are, the slower our metabolic rate becomes. In general, our activity declines as we progress in age. There are many factors that are to blame for this, but probably the two most significant are our employment and urban lifestyle. Thus we see that our resting metabolism is not constant, but can increase or decrease depending on our food choices and the use of our skeletal muscle.

In summary, the two main hormones that control our resting metabolic rate are insulin and thyroxine. Insulin regulates what type of energy we use at any give time. Carbohydrates are used when blood insulin levels are elevated, while fatty acids are released from fat cells when insulin is low. Thyroxine regulates how much energy is expended daily. How this hormone works is not completely elucidated. Fortunately, the level of both hormones can be influenced by other risk factors. Insulin levels can be effected by the Food Selection Risk factor while thyroxine can be effected by the Physical Activity Risk factor. For most of us our resting metabolic rate is the predominant source involved in energy expenditure. This amounts to eighty to eighty-five percent of the total energy expended in a day. The exception to this are elite athletes who expend an additional twenty-five to thirty percent by participating in moderate-high intensity training. Our skeletal muscle consumes the most energy while at rest compared to any other organ system. The use or disuse of skeletal muscle can directly effect our resting metabolic rate.

Chapter 11

The Fat Utility Risk factor is a simple way to explain why some of us gain more fat pound than others, despite having approximately equal caloric intake or Food Selection and Stress Risks, and caloric expenditure or Physical Activity and Metabolism Risks. Fat Utility is also the predominant reason why we are unable to keep weight off for any extended period, say one year. Importantly, in order to change Fat Utility, we must recognize that it is independent of caloric intake and expenditure. This risk factor may make it seem impossible for some of us to keep weight off, because we may store the small amount of fat we consumed extremely efficient. Hence, only minuscule amounts of fat can reflect large gains in fatty acid absorption into our fat cells.

Fat Utility in action can be easy to identify in the early stage of our development such as childhood. For instance, everybody has seen an extremely heavy ten year old before, and wondered what the parents are feeding this kid. Certainly, if our social beliefs have anything to do with knowledge, then we are truly lacking in knowledge when it comes to the subject of fat. Of course this child will eventually over consume by increasing episodes of binge eating. But this behavior typically presents itself after the child is over weight, and parallels the same time he or she begins to feel different from their peers. The internal stimuli, anxiety, is thought to propagate internal conflict, which can result in a binge disorder and can be very difficult to modify.

In addition to over consumption of food, we also recognize that these children have environmental factors that are considered to promote continued weight gain. That is, they will typically have parents or sibling who are also over weight, and their behaviors may eventually be assimilated by the child. But, the assertion of the Risk Factor Theory is that these problems are only manifestations of this underlying risk factor, Fat Utility. The association between the child's obese nature and the parents or siblings body habitus is nothing more than the existence of having a similar genetic makeup. This means that the greatest risk each of us has for gaining weight depends on whether or not our parents are over weight.

In support of this theory, recent evidence suggests that the caloric intake and dietary composition between obese children and adolescents, and their non obese counterparts are very similar. In addition, the two groups have been shown to have only minimal differences in metabolic rate and physical activity. Other compelling evidence comes from recent studies on fat blocking medications. In general, medications that target this risk factor do not cause rapid weight loss, but are shown to be effective in keeping weight off once it is lost. This is very significant. Potential fat genes have also been identified.

However, more often this phenomenon is

expressed after puberty, and is usually less dramatic. Hence, when and how severe we develop this fat trait depends on our fate genes. Furthermore, there is likely more that a single gene responsible for the expression of Fat Utility. Physical signs of increased fat pounds may not appear until we are in our young adult life or after pregnancy, and may initially go unrecognized until we have put on twenty or more extra pounds.

This risk factor has two main components to its overall effect. Fat Utility can be defined as the amount of fatty acids that our body will allow to cross our digestive lining out of the total amount we consume and the amount and ease in which our body can store fatty acids into fat cells. The ability our body has to release fatty acids that are stored in fat cells is thought to be related to our level of carbohydrate storage.

Once fatty acids are consumed then a variety of factors which effect the amount that actually gets absorbed through the gut lining. This is because the biological processes involved are somewhat complicated , and rely on multiple organs in order to be fulfilled. Simplistically, fatty acids have to be package so that they can be soluble in water, which in turn allows them to get near our digestive lining, and be transferred across. This process is called emulsification. The liver, pancreas, and biliary ductal systems influence the amount of fatty acids that are emulsified and subsequently activated, which enable them to cross our digestive lining. In addition, the rate of motility of our gastrointestinal system and structure of the digestive lining, can also effect the amount of fatty acids absorbed. As such, this area has been targeted by medical research as a viable way to effect the amount of fatty acids that can get through the gut and be deposited into fat cells. Importantly, nondigestible fiber found in fruits and vegetables will also decrease the amount of fat that passes through the digestive lining. Nondigestible fiber can physically block fat and also increase digestive motility.

There may be great variability from person to person, in the amount of fat that can cross our digestive lining because, this process is effected by many organs systems. For instance, the enzymatic activity of our pancreatic lipase enzymes can directly influence the sensitivity of the emulsified fatty acids receptiveness through our digestive lining. Also, the amount of bile our liver secretes relates to how much fatty acid can be emulsified and made available for transport. In addition, the rate of motility of our digestive tract effects the ability for the above systems to get their job done within an allotted time. All three of these organ systems may function slightly different in all of us which may effect how much fat we retain. Structural variability in the digestive lining is considered a medical disorder and is therefore not discussed here.

Once fatty acids are transported through the gut, they pass through our lymphatic system in a packaged particle, called a chylomicron. This large cluster of fatty acids are then predominantly sent to peripheral tissues to be utilized as energy by our muscle, heart, and kidneys, and subsequently to our fat cells, to stored some of the remaining fatty acids. How receptive these tissues are to the fatty acids is related to the energetic needs of our body at any given time. Under normal situations, after the feeding of the muscle, heart, and kidneys there are still plenty of fatty acids left over for our fat cells to indulge. How receptive our fat cells are to more fatty acid absorption is likely, however, to be dependent on the individual and his or her genetic make up. This may also be true for skeletal muscle. Consequently, the amount of fatty acids that are absorbed by fat cells may differ significantly between individuals, and does not reflect our metabolic state. After the chylomicrom has passed through these organ systems not all of the fatty acids are removed. It is then transported to the liver where it may be utilized in a variety of ways depending on the liver's need, as well as, its perception of the body's needs. Effecting the amount of fatty acids that are actually absorbed through t he gut lining indirectly effects the amount stored in fat cells. By the time the chylomicron gets to the fat cells there is very little left over for them.

When fatty acids become stored in fat cells, this theory becomes more complex because fatty acids are continually being released and absorbed by fat cells to facilitate our resting metabolism. Interestingly, the release of fatty acids follow a completely different pathway than the absorption of fatty acids. As a matter of fact, the two pathways package fatty acids differently. Therefore, the fatty acids represent two distinct pools. Fat storage is actually the difference between the total amount of fat absorbed, and the total amount of fat released by fat cells. For most of us, the equilibrium between the two pathways tend to favor the fat storage side. Unfortunately, most of us experience an incremental increase in fat storage daily. However, from the perspective of our body, fat storage is what it strives to achieve. This means that once the fat is stored in fat cells, our body will desire to keep it there. Only when it is absolutely necessary will we release more fatty acids than what we store.

In summary, Fat Utility Risk is independent of how many calories we consume or expend, but depends on our genetic make-up. The number one risk in becoming over weight is whether or not our parents are over weight. Over consumption and environmental factors are considered to be late manifestations of this risk factor, and not the underlying cause of obesity. Importantly, nondigestible fiber found in fruits and vegetables can decrease the amount of fat that is actually transported through the digestive lining. This ultimately affects the amount of fatty acids that can get stored in fat cells.

Chapter 12

As mentioned in the introduction, the Food Selection Risk factor has an overwhelming impact on our weight loss, and especially weight gain. This factor is so strong that it can influence the Stress, Metabolism, and Fat Utility Risk factors. Just by changing our food selections and when we eat certain food groups we can actually manipulate four of the five risk factors. An ideal diet from the perspective of weight loss should therefore fulfill the following criteria by increasing the occurrence of fatty acid and protein used to run our metabolism, decrease the occurrence of eating when food is available or when we are not hungry, allow us to use more energy during resting states, and decrease the amount of fat that actually gets absorbed by the digestive tract.

An argument can be made that we are what we eat. This adage deviates a bit when we take in to consideration longevity. For instance, there are only minor caloric differences between a saturated, trans, mono-unsaturated, or polyunsaturated fatty acid. They are all roughly nine calories per gram and so they are equal. From a longevity perspective, however, trans and saturated fatty acids increase cardiovascular and cancer risks, while polyunsaturated and mono-unsaturated may provide cardiovascular protection. Similarly with carbohydrates, their caloric contribution is four calories per gram. Yet, carbohydrate products that contain antioxidants and fiber have been shown to decrease many forms of cancer and other chronic disease states, such as diabetes and cardiovascular disease. Thus, an ideal diet should also include food groups that are know to extend our longevity.

The Cycle Diet is designed to emulate the above principles. In addition, the Food Selection Risk is used to minimize the effects of other Risk Factors that weight loss sets off. We can effect the Food Selection Risk factor in a positive way by either reducing the caloric consumption or change the type of caloric food groups we chose to consume. Severe caloric restriction or below thirteen hundred calories a day will escalate the Stress and slow the Metabolism Risk factors and likely result in weight gain. On the other hand, by selecting certain food types we can produce weight loss without adversely effecting other risks. This strategy also includes what time of day in which we consume certain food groups. For example, the optimal time to consume carbohydrate or fat food groups in the morning or early afternoon. This assures ourselves that these foods will be used as expended energy instead of glycogen or fat storage.

The Food Selection Risk can effect the Stress Risk which is typically instrumental in rapid weight gain. More importantly, the negative impact Stress has on us when we try to lose weight by caloric restriction is one underlying reason why we will discontinue a diet. There are only two ways in which we can effect the Stress Risk in a positive way. The first is by prescription medication and the second is to incorporate carbohydrate and fat combination food into our diet regimen. Remember, the inherent positive reward system we have built in us is there for a reason and will not go away. The trick however is to appease this system so that we can have some control over it.

Food Selection can also effect our risk factor Metabolism either in a positive or negative way. Of course we desire to influence Metabolism in a positive way and the only way we can do this without medication or exercise is to substitute protein calories for carbohydrate calories. Remember in Chapter Four, we discussed the fact that carbohydrates in the form of glucose are essential for certain vital organs, such as our brain adrenal gland, and red blood cells. When we use fats or fatty acids as a source of energy, we are also using protein. Protein can be converted into glucose, or a glucose intermediate where as cat cannot. This conversion, protein to glucose actually effects our metabolism in a positive way. However, we have to make our body use this system, because if it perceives that carbohydrates are available then there is no way we will use protein, and subsequently fat as an energy source.

Substituting proteins for carbohydrates will eventually result in the complete depletion of carbohydrates. We do not like this for long periods of time because a gradual increase in blood nitrogen will result. Our brain will reluctantly begin to use an energy source termed ketones. This is absolutely not necessary for efficient use of fatty acids as a source of energy. As a matter of fact, the rate that fatty acids are used as energy is only minimally different during prolonged periods of carbohydrate depletion, compared to the initial stages. However, the amount of ketones and nitrogen in our blood is drastically different.

By selecting food groups that are high in dietary and nondigestible fibers, we can also effect the Fat Utility Risk factor. This is important because it will allow us to continue to consume food products that taste good without receiving the full caloric impact. We may recall that nondigestible fibers found in specific vegetables can decrease the amount of fat that actually gets absorbed through the gut lining, by acting as a physical blocker and by increasing our gut motility. Dietary fiber found in vegetables can decrease the amount of fat that actually gets absorbed through the gut lining, by acting as a physical blocker and by increasing our gut motility. Dietary fiber found in vegetables is also important because it can slow the rate of carbohydrate absorption through the gut lining. Ultimately, this is beneficial because these fibers slow carbohydrate storage, which in turn, keeps the rate of fat storage to a minimum.

Chapter 13

The Cycle Diet consists of four stages. Each stage is designed specifically to minimize our Five Risk Factors that cause weight gain and maximize our longevity by decreasing our chance for chronic disease states such as cardiovascular disease, diabetes, and cancer. One complete cycle takes eleven days. The first stage or Stage One is six days, Stage Two is one day, Stage Three is three days, and Stage Four is one day. After Stage Four we repeat the cycle again and can be used safely and effectively until you reach your desired weight.

Stage One lasts for six days and is designed to reduce our carbohydrate storage or glycogen, especially in the evening hours. By doing this we are actually changing our metabolic state from glucose expenditure and fat storage to protein and fat expenditure a few hours prior to waking up.
Breakfast: Drink one 8 ounce glass of water immediately before meal. Contrary to popular belief, you may skip breakfast and go to the snack selection or lunch within four hours after getting out of bed. If you are not hungry then do not eat breakfast, because this is clearly the time of the day in which we are most efficient at burning fat.
Select one of the following six listed below.
1. One serving of a hot or cold cereal that contains whole grain wheat, brown rice, oat, and or

bran which consists of less than forty grams of carbohydrates and two grams of fat. Non fat or one percent milk. Sugar substitute maybe added. Coffee.

2. Two slices of bread or toast that contain wheat, oat, and or bran consisting of no more that 15 grams of carbohydrates and 1 gram of fat per slice. No more than one teaspoon of margarine type spread that is made predominately with soybean or canola oil. Black or green tea, or coffee. Sugar substitute. Non fat or one percent milk may be added to coffee only.

3. One bagel or muffin that contains wheat, oat, and or bran consisting of no more than forty grams of carbohydrates and 2 grams of fat. No more than one teaspoon of low fat cream cheese spread or soybean or canola spread. Black or green tea, or coffee. Sugar substitute if desired. Non fat or one percent milk may be added to coffee only.

4. Three or less of the following whole fresh fruits: apple, orange, peach, banana. No more than one watercress, cantaloupe,, grapefruit, or no more that fifty grapes. Do not puree or blend. Black or green tea, or coffee. Sugar substitute if desired. Dairy products inactivate the antioxidants in fruit, and black or green tea.

5. One small ten ounce bowl of low or no fat yogurt which consists of no more than thirty grams of carbohydrates and two grams of fat. One of the following fresh fruits, apple, peach , fifteen grapes, grapefruit, or one half watercress or cantaloupe. Black or green tea or coffee without milk. Sugar substitute if desired.

6. Two eggs scrambled or fried with one teaspoon canola oil. One slice of wheat, oat, and or bran toast without spread. Coffee, black or green tea. Low fat or one percent milk may be added to coffee only. Sugar substitute if desired. Male participants can select this menu on two of the six days while females can select it three of the six days.

Snack: Before lunch you may snack on carrot or celery sticks or cucumber slices without added salt. You may drink one diet soda or unlimited ice tea with lemon slices. No sugar substitute.

Lunch: Eat at least four hours after you get out of bed Drink one eight ounce glass of water immediately before your sandwich meal only. You may select salad and soup for three of the days or you can select a salad two days, soup two days, and sandwich two days. Do not skip lunch.

Select one of the following three below.

1. Salad may include generous amounts of iceberg lettuce, cabbage, celery, carrots, cucumber, bell pepper, corn, peas, and or onion. You may add one hard boiled egg. If desired a generous portion of chicken, turkey or low sodium and low fat ham. Dressing must contain less than thirty grams carbohydrates and less than three grams of fat or low fat vinaigrette. Ice tea or non fat milk if desired.

2. Soup may either be from a can or from the recipe list found in the Appendix. No more than two twenty ounce bowls of low sodium or three hundred micrograms (mg) or less per twenty ounces of vegetable, chicken and vegetable, turkey and

vegetable. No more than three twenty ounce bowls from the recipe list which includes vegetable, chicken or beef and vegetable, basque, bean and tomato, chicken, beef, fish and shrimp soups. Three low sodium backed crackers per bowl may be added to the chicken, beef, fish or shrimp soups. Ice tea or non fat milk if desired.

3. One sandwich that includes two slices of oat, wheat, and or bran bread that may be toasted. At least one of the following vegetables should be added to the sandwich, lettuce, tomato, dill pickles, or onion. Generous amounts of chicken breast, roast beef, turkey, canned tuna or chicken packed in water not oil. Mustard, one tablespoon of low fat mayonnaise, and pepper are optional. Ice tea or non fat milk if desired.

Snack: if desired you may snack on the same items as morning snack.

Dinner: Two eight ounce glasses of water immediately before meal. You may select one of the three meats plus one vegetable or salad dish. For those of us who do not eat meat, no more than two twenty ounce bowls of a vegetable, basque, or bean and tomato soup may be substituted. Cooking preparation for the following meat selections are included below. Generous portions of both food items are allowed. The majority of the vegetables or salad should be consumed after your meat selection. By doing this, we are considering the different digestive rates of food items. Optimal time for dinner consumption is two or more hours before bedtime.

73

Select one of the following three below.

1. Beef includes eye of round, toploin, tenderloin, sirloin, and tritip. They may be slow cooked in a crock pot with water and low sodium seasoning or broth, barbecued, boiled, or stir fry. Can be marinated in Worcestershire sauce for two or more hours in the refrigerator. No more than one quarter cup of barbecue sauce may be brushed on meat prior to cooking. Stir fry technique requires browning slicked meat in two teaspoons of canola or olive oil per pound of meat or poultry then adding one quarter cup of water per pound to saute for one minute, then drain and add desired vegetables from vegetable list below. Two tablespoons of steak sauce is optional.

2. Chicken can be slow cooked in water and low sodium seasoning or broth, barbecued, broiled, slow baked in a bag with onions and garlic, or stir fried. It may be cooked with skin intact but must be removed prior to consuming. Barbecue sauce should be added prior to barbecuing. Studies have shown that this technique decreases carcinogens during barbecuing. Use same stir fry technique as beef

3. White fillet fish only so ask your butcher. May be grilled or slow baked in a bag with low sodium seasoning, onions, and minced garlic if desired.

Select one of the following two below.

1. Vegetables include green beans fresh or in a can, corn on the cob or low sodium corn in a can. Steamed broccoli, green beans, asparagus, cabbage, and carrots are preferred. Generous portions are

allowed. Served with pepper and lemon juice if desired but do not add salt.

2. Salad as described in the above lunch section.

Stage Two is for one day and is considered a diet break. Food Selection is consequently more pleasing to our taste. The carbohydrate and fat combinations will also transiently elevate our serotonin levels. One of the three meals maybe purchased at a restaurant as take out. Avoid snacking between meals.

Breakfast: Two eight ounce glasses of water immediately before meal. Optional food items that are underlined do not have to be include in the meal and should be consumed after the non optional items.

Select one of the four following items below.

1. One twenty ounce bowl of any hot or cold cereal with one teaspoon of sugar if desired. One of the following fresh fruits, apple, orange, grapefruit, cantaloupe, thirty grapes, or watercress. Coffee, black or green tea. Optional includes one slice of whole wheat, bran and or oat bread or toast with one teaspoon of canola spread if desired. No more than eight ounces of one or two percent milk may be added.

2. No more than three medium size of eight inch diameter pancakes of your choice or no more than two french toasts. One of the following fresh fruits, apple, orange, grapefruit, cantaloupe, thirty grapes, or watercress. One eighth of a cup of any syrup, jelly or fruit preserve. Coffee, black or green tea. Optional includes no more than eight ounces of one or two

percent milk.

3. Two eggs made scrambled, fried in one teaspoon of canola, hard boiled or poached. One medium serving of hash brown potatoes fried in nonfat canola no stick cooking spray. Coffee, black or green tea. One or two percent milk may be added to coffee and one teaspoon of sugar may be added. Optional includes one slice of whole wheat, bran and or oat bread or toast without spread. Optional includes one of the following fresh fruits, apple, orange, grapefruit, cantaloupe, thirty grapes, or watercress.

4. Three egg or less ham omelet without cheese. Two slices of whole wheat, bran and or oat bread without spread. No more than two of the following fresh fruits, apple, orange, grapefruit, cantaloupe, thirty grapes, or watercress. Coffee, black or green tea. One teaspoon of sugar may be added.

Lunch: Two eight ounce glasses of water immediately before your meal. The salad should be prepared with only the ingredients listed on salad preparation in Stage One. Each lunch must have a salad with the main meal shown in bold. Optional food items underlined do not have to be included in the meal, and should be consumed after the main meal and salad. Optional drink item can be ingested at any time during the meal.

Select one of the following five items shown below.

1. No more than two grilled chicken sandwiches of your choice without cheese, mayonnaise, or house sauce. Two of the following fresh fruits, apple,

76

orange, grapefruit, cantaloupe, thirty grapes or watercress. One small twelve ounce bowl salad with choice of dressing of one tablespoon. Optional food items of no more than ten chips of your choice without dip. Optional 12 ounce ice tea or diet soda.

2. No more than two ham or roast beef with white cheese sandwiches. Bread should be made from whole wheat, bran and or oat bread. One tablespoon of any mayonnaise may be added. Lettuce, tomato and pickles should be added. One of the following fresh fruits, apple, orange, grapefruit, cantaloupe, thirty grapes or watercress. One small twelve ounce bowl salad with one tablespoon of your choice salad dressing. Optional food items of no more than ten chips of your choice without dip. Optional 12 ounce ice tea or diet soda.

3. No more than two single hamburgers cooked any way but with most of the animal grease removed. Whole wheat, oat, or bran bun bread are preferable to enriched hamburger buns. Fresh lettuce, tomato, and onion should be included. This provides nondigestible fiber that blocks fat absorption. One tablespoon of catsup, or any type of mustard may be added but no mayonnaise or house sauce. One small twelve ounce bowl of salad with one tablespoon of your choice of salad dressing. Optional food include small portion of french fries of less than twelve or hash browns of one quarter dinner size plate with one tablespoon of catsup. No additional salt should be added. Optional 12 ounce ice tea or diet soda.

4. No more than two bean burritos or chicken and

black bean soft tacos without cheese. Corn or flour tortillas. Fresh lettuce, tomato, one quarter of avocado but not guacamole and or onion should be included. Liberal amounts of salsa or hot sauce can be added. One small twelve ounce bowl salad with one tablespoon of your choice salad dressing. Optional food items of no more than ten chips of your choice without dip. Do not add cheese, sour cream, salt, or guacamole. Optional 12 ounce ice tea or diet soda.

5. No more than two medium slices of pizza of your choice. One small twelve ounce bowl salad with one tablespoon of your choice of salad dressing. Optional 12 ounce ice tea or diet soda.

Dinner: Drink two glasses of water immediately after entire meal. Salad is prepared only with the ingredients listed in Stage One. Salad must accompany main meal shown below. Optional food items do not have to be consumed if you are not hungry. Optional beverage may be consumed at any time during the meal.

Select one of the following five items shown below.

1. No more than two chicken fajitas. Two flour tortillas only. Sauteed onions and or green peppers may be added. Fresh lettuce, tomato, onion, and peppers should be added. You may add one tablespoon of low fat cheese, low fat sour cream, or low fat guacamole. One small twelve ounce bowl salad with one tablespoon of your choice of salad dressing. Optional items include one cup of brown

rice, or black beans, or fat free refried beans. Optional items include five chips with or without salsa. Optional beverage includes ice tea, diet soda, or one glass of wine. Optional dessert includes no more than two three ounce portions of any fat free pastry. Remember two eight ounce glasses of water immediately after entire meal.

2. Steamed crab or lobster dipped in no more than one quarter cup of low fat mayonnaise and or one quarter cup of seafood sauce. Fresh squeezed lemon juice may be added. Cajun or other spices may be added to dip sauce. One small twelve ounce bowl salad with one tablespoon of your choice of salad dressing. Generous portion of steamed or sauteed fresh green beans, carrots, asparagus, artichoke, pea pods. Optional beverage includes ice tea, diet soda, or one glass of wine. Optional dessert includes no more than two three ounce portions of any fat free pastry. Remember two eight ounce glasses of water immediately after entire meal.

3. Stir fried shrimp in garlic sauce and fresh vegetables. Fresh vegetables can include green beans pea pods, and others. One small twelve ounce bowl salad with one tablespoon of your choice of salad dressing. Optional item includes no more than two slices of bread of your choice with one teaspoon of canola or garlic spread. Optional beverage includes ice tea, diet soda, or one glass of wine. Optional dessert includes no more than two three ounce portions of any fat free pastry. Remember two eight ounce glasses of water immediately after entire meal.

4. No more than two generous portions of spaghetti with tomato sauce or meat and tomato sauce. If hamburger is used then drain animal fat after browning. One small twelve ounce bowl salad with one tablespoon of your choice of salad dressing. Optional item includes no more than two slices of bread of your choice with one teaspoon of canola or garlic spread. Optional beverage includes ice tea, diet soda, or one glass of wine. Optional dessert includes no more than two three ounce portions of any fat free pastry. Remember two eight ounce glasses of water immediately after entire meal.

5. Any of the food items listed in morning or lunch menus for Stage Two above.

Stage Three of The Cycle Diet lasts for three days and is designed to be caloric restrictive. We should make a strong attempt to adhere to the diet for all three days. Lunch and dinner comprise almost entirely of a soup diet.

Breakfast: Drink one eight ounce glass of water immediately before meal. Your may skip breakfast but not the water.. If you are not hungry then do not eat breakfast.

Select from the six breakfast selections below.

1. One serving of a hot or cold cereal that contains whole grain wheat, brown rice, oat, and or bran which consists of less than forty grams of carbohydrates and two grams of fat. Non fat or one percent milk. Sugar substitute maybe added. Coffee.

2. Two slices of bread or toast that contain wheat,

oat, and or bran consisting of no more that 15 grams of carbohydrates and 1 gram of fat per slice. No more than one teaspoon of margarine type spread that is made predominately with soybean or canola oil. Black or green tea, or coffee. Sugar substitute. Non fat or one percent milk may be added to coffee only.

3. One bagel or muffin that contains wheat, oat, and or bran consisting of no more than forty grams of carbohydrates and 2 grams of fat. No more than one teaspoon of low fat cream cheese spread or soybean or canola spread. Black or green tea, or coffee. Sugar substitute if desired. Non fat or one percent milk may be added to coffee only.

4. Three or less of the following whole fresh fruits: apple, orange, peach, banana. No more than one watercress, cantaloupe,, grapefruit, or no more that fifty grapes. Do not puree or blend. Black or green tea, or coffee. Sugar substitute if desired. Dairy products inactivate the antioxidants in fruit, and black or green tea.

5. One small ten ounce bowl of low or no fat yogurt which consists of no more than thiry grams of carbohydrates and two grams of fat. One of the following fresh fruits, apple, peach , fifteen grapes, grapefruit, or one half watercress or cantaloupe. Black or green tea or coffee without milk. Sugar substitute if desired.

6. Two eggs scrambled or fried with one teaspoon canola oil. One slice of wheat, oat, and or bran toast without spread. Coffee, black or green tea. Low fat or one percent milk may be added to coffee

only. Sugar substitute if desired. Snack: Before lunch you may snack on carrot and celery sticks, or cucumber slices without added salt. You may drink one diet soda or unlimited ice tea with slices. No sugar or sugar substitute.

Lunch: Do not skip. Eat this meal at least four hours after waking up. You may want to make large amounts of soup at one time so that it will last for a few days. No required water consumption. Soup may either be from a can or from the recipe list found in the Appendix. No more than two twenty ounce bowls of low sodium or three hundred micrograms (mg) or less per twenty ounces of vegetable, chicken and vegetable, turkey and vegetable. No more than three twenty ounce bowls from the recipe list which includes vegetable, chicken or beef and vegetable, basque, bean and tomato, chicken, beef, fish and shrimp soups. Three low sodium backed crackers per bowl may be added to the chicken, beef, fish or shrimp soups. Ice tea or non fat milk if desired. Snack: None.

Dinner: Includes no more than three servings of any of the soup selections plus one serving of salad. Salad may include 12 ounces total of iceberg lettuce, cabbage, celery, carrots, cucumber, bell pepper, corn, peas, and or onion. You may add hard boiled egg. If desired a portion of chicken, turkey or low sodium and low fat ham. Dressing must contain less than thirty grams carbohydrates and less than three grams of fat or low fat vinaigrette. Optimal time for consumption is two or more hours before bedtime.

No water requirements prior or after meal. Optional beverage includes one eight ounce non-caffeinated diet soda or one percent eight ounce glass of milk.

Stage Four lasts for one day and is designed to elevate serotonin levels. This stage will effectively reduce the Stress Risk factor which may have elevated after Stage Three. One of the three meals maybe purchased at a restaurant as take out. Avoid snacking between meals.

Breakfast: Two eight ounce glasses of water immediately before meal. Optional food items that are underlined do not have to be include in the meal and should be consumed after the non optional items.

Select one of the four following items below.

1. One twenty ounce bowl of any hot or cold cereal with one teaspoon of sugar if desired. One of the following fresh fruits, apple, orange, grapefruit, cantaloupe, thirty grapes, or watercress. Coffee, black or green tea. Optional includes one slice of whole wheat, bran and or oat bread or toast with one teaspoon of canola spread if desired. No more than eight ounces of one or two percent milk may be added.

2. No more than three medium size of eight inch diameter pancakes of your choice or no more than two french toasts. One of the following fresh fruits, apple, orange, grapefruit, cantaloupe, thirty grapes, or watercress. One eighth of a cup of any syrup, jelly or fruit preserve. Coffee, black or green tea. Optional includes no more than eight ounces of one or two

percent milk.

3. Two eggs made scrambled, fried in one teaspoon of canola, hard boiled or poached. One medium serving of hash brown potatoes fried in nonfat canola no stick cooking spray. Coffee, black or green tea. One or two percent milk may be added to coffee and one teaspoon of sugar may be added. Optional includes one slice of whole wheat, bran and or oat bread or toast without spread. Optional includes one of the following fresh fruits, apple, orange, grapefruit, cantaloupe, thirty grapes, or watercress.

4. Three egg or less ham omelet without cheese. Two slices of whole wheat, bran and or oat bread without spread. No more than two of the following fresh fruits, apple, orange, grapefruit, cantaloupe, thirty grapes, or watercress. Coffee, black or green tea. One teaspoon of sugar may be added.

Lunch: Two eight ounce glasses of water immediately before your meal. The salad should be prepared with only the ingredients listed on salad preparation in Stage One. Each lunch must have a salad with the main meal shown in bold. Optional food items underlined do not have to be included in the meal, and should be consumed after the main meal and salad. Optional drink item can be ingested at any time during the meal.

Select one of the following five items shown below.

1. No more than two grilled chicken sandwiches of your choice without cheese, mayonnaise, or house sauce. Two of the following fresh fruits, apple,

orange, grapefruit, cantaloupe, thirty grapes or watercress. One small twelve ounce bowl salad with choice of dressing of one tablespoon. Optional food items of no more than ten chips of your choice without dip. Optional 12 ounce ice tea or diet soda.

2. No more than two ham or roast beef with white cheese sandwiches. Bread should be made from whole wheat, bran and or oat bread. One tablespoon of any mayonnaise may be added. Lettuce, tomato and pickles should be added. One of the following fresh fruits, apple, orange, grapefruit, cantaloupe, thirty grapes or watercress. One small twelve ounce bowl salad with one tablespoon of your choice salad dressing. Optional food items of no more than ten chips of your choice without dip. Optional 12 ounce ice tea or diet soda.

3. No more than two single hamburgers cooked any way but with most of the animal grease removed. Whole wheat, oat, or bran bun bread are preferable to enriched hamburger buns. Fresh lettuce, tomato, and onion should be included. This provides nondigestible fiber that blocks fat absorption. One tablespoon of catsup, or any type of mustard may be added but no mayonnaise or house sauce. One small twelve ounce bowl of salad with one tablespoon of your choice of salad dressing. Optional food include small portion of french fries of less than twelve or hash browns of one quarter dinner size plate with one tablespoon of catsup. No additional salt should be added. Optional 12 ounce ice tea or diet soda.

4. No more than two bean burritos or chicken and

black bean soft tacos without cheese. Corn or flour tortillas. Fresh lettuce, tomato, one quarter of avocado but not guacamole and or onion should be included. Liberal amounts of salsa or hot sauce can be added. One small twelve ounce bowl salad with one tablespoon of your choice salad dressing. Optional food items of no more than ten chips of your choice without dip. Do not add cheese, sour cream, salt, or guacamole. Optional 12 ounce ice tea or diet soda.

5. No more than two medium slices of pizza of your choice. One small twelve ounce bowl salad with one tablespoon of your choice of salad dressing. Optional 12 ounce ice tea or diet soda.

Dinner: Drink two glasses of water immediately after entire meal. Salad is prepared only with the ingredients listed in Stage One. Salad must accompany main meal shown below. Optional food items do not have to be consumed if you are not hungry. Optional beverage may be consumed at any time during the meal.

Select one of the following five items shown below.

1. No more than two chicken fajitas. Two flour tortillas only. Sauteed onions and or green peppers may be added. Fresh lettuce, tomato, onion, and peppers should be added. You may add one tablespoon of low fat cheese, low fat sour cream, or low fat guacamole. One small twelve ounce bowl salad with one tablespoon of your choice of salad dressing. Optional items include one cup of brown

rice, or black beans, or fat free refried beans. Optional items include five chips with or without salsa. Optional beverage includes ice tea, diet soda, or one glass of wine. Optional dessert includes no more than two three ounce portions of any fat free pastry. Remember two eight ounce glasses of water immediately after entire meal.

2. Steamed crab or lobster dipped in no more than one quarter cup of low fat mayonnaise and or one quarter cup of seafood sauce. Fresh squeezed lemon juice may be added. Cajun or other spices may be added to dip sauce. One small twelve ounce bowl salad with one tablespoon of your choice of salad dressing. Generous portion of steamed or sauteed fresh green beans, carrots, asparagus, artichoke, pea pods. Optional beverage includes ice tea, diet soda, or one glass of wine. Optional dessert includes no more than two three ounce portions of any fat free pastry. Remember two eight ounce glasses of water immediately after entire meal.

3. Stir fried shrimp in garlic sauce and fresh vegetables. Fresh vegetables can include green beans pea pods, and others. One small twelve ounce bowl salad with one tablespoon of your choice of salad dressing. Optional item includes no more than two slices of bread of your choice with one teaspoon of canola or garlic spread. Optional beverage includes ice tea, diet soda, or one glass of wine. Optional dessert includes no more than two three ounce portions of any fat free pastry. Remember two eight ounce glasses of water immediately after entire meal.

4. No more than two generous portions of spaghetti with tomato sauce or meat and tomato sauce. If hamburger is used then drain animal fat after browning. One small twelve ounce bowl salad with one tablespoon of your choice of salad dressing. Optional item includes no more than two slices of bread of your choice with one teaspoon of canola or garlic spread. Optional beverage includes ice tea, diet soda, or one glass of wine. Optional dessert includes no more than two three ounce portions of any fat free pastry. Remember two eight ounce glasses of water immediately after entire meal.

5. Any of the food items listed in morning or lunch menus for Stage Four above.

At the end of Stage Four, we have completed one full cycle of The Cycle Diet and are ready to start Stage One again on day twelve of the diet. For maximum results, The Cycle Diet should be repeated at least four to six times or approximately two months. Once youre desired weight is attained, you may want to stay on the diet but maintain your weight. In this situation, you can decrease the duration of Stages One and Three. For increased weight loss, you can lengthen the duration of Stages One and Three to a maximum of ten and five days respectively.

Chapter 14

Since our goal is to minimize all five risk factors that cause weight gain, we need to minimize our Physical Activity Risk factor as well. As mentioned in previous chapters, the Physical Activity Risk can positively effect Metabolism and Stress Risks. It can however indirectly has an adverse effect on Food Selection Risk because our metabolism increases which signals increased caloric consumption. In addition, thirty minutes of moderate activity a day improves other longevity markers such as smoking, high blood pressure, high cholesterol, cardiovascular disease, and diabetes. What is important to understand is that the thirty minutes of activity a day can be accumulated. This means that four to six five-minute separate bouts of activity is all we need daily. To fulfill The Cycle Program requirements, you must maintain at least four separate five-minute bouts of activity a day while on The Cycle Diet.

Below is a list of acceptable activities to help you determine the amount of physical activity you are getting per week, Table One. You may also want to write down your activities for approximately two weeks. This will assist you in determining if the Physical Activity Risk factor is impeding your weight loss goals. It is important for you to not under estimate the amount of actual walking you do. We recommend at least three of the four separate five - minute bouts of physical activity to be walking with a gradual progression to brisk walking. A pedometer can be purchased for under fifty dollars at your nearest sporting good store, and will give a good estimate of how many miles you actually walk. Using this method, approximately one and one half to two miles a day of non-continuous walking will sufficiently minimize the Physical Activity Risk factor.

Table One: List of acceptable physical activities. All activities should be five or more minutes of continuous activity.

vacuuming	sweeping	mopping
cleaning windows	cleaning counter tops	
carrying an infant	moving furniture	
washing the car	shopping	
cleaning the garage	bike riding	
roller skating	tennis	walking
golf	home repairs	gardening

In addition to the above physical activities, we recommend that you participate in two separate episodes of resistance activity that lasts for at least two minutes. You may select from walking up and down stairs, traditional, knee, or wall push-ups, or sit-ups Those of us who are currently sedentary, minimally active, or presently taking prescription medication should consult your primary care physician for advise before initiating this program.

The Cycle Program can achieve a positive influence on all of the five risk factors that affect weight loss. The projected amount of weight loss will progress to about one percent of your total body weight per week by the second month of continuous participation of The Cycle Program. This is considered the maximum limits for medically unsupervised weight loss.

Appendix

Selected Soup Recipes

1. <u>Vegetable Soup</u>: Add one cup water and three 15 ounce low sodium low fat beef or chicken broth to large soup pot. Add fress potato cubes from two medium potatoes, one medium onion chopped, one cup corn*, one cup sliced carrots, one cup sliced celery, one cp shelled green peas and green beans*. Add one sixteen ounce can undrained whole tomatoes if beef broth is used. Heat to near boil than reduce heat and simmer 45 minutes or until vegetables are tender.

2. <u>Chicken or Beef Vegetable Soup</u>: One to two pounds of boneless Chicken breast or select cut Beef that is eye of round, toploin, tenderloin, sirloin, tritip may be boiled or browned with non fat no stick cooking spray or water. In separate soup pot, add two cups water, two 15 ounce cans of low sodium low fat chicken or beef broth, one chopped onion, one cup chopped green peppers, one cup corn*, one cup sliced carrots. Shred or slice the chicken or beef and add to soup. Add low sodium garlic salt and pepper to taste. Simmer or slow cook in crock pot for two to three hours. Skim top residue every hour.

3. <u>Basque soup</u>: Add one cup water and two 15 ounce cans low fat low sodium chicken broth to large soup pot. Add three quarters bead of chopped cabbage, two minced cloves of garlic, one medium chopped onion, and cup sliced carrots, two sixteen ounce cans undrained Italian whole tomatoes to pot. Simmer or

slow cook for 45 minutes or until vegetables tender. Add low sodium garlic salt and pepper to taste while simmering.

4. <u>Bean and Tomato</u>: Add eight cups of water to two cups of kidney or pinto beans and bring to boil then simmer in large pot for two to three hours until tender. Drain water leaving beans in pot. Then add two 16-ounce cans crushed tomatoes which maybe seasoned but less than 300mg of sodium per can, two cups water, one forth cup of brown rice, one cup corn*, fresh onion. Add low sodium garlic salt and pepper to taste while simmering while covered for 45 minutes. Additional water may be added for desired consistency.

5. <u>Chicken** and Tomato:</u> Add one 16 ounce can diced tomatoes, two 16 ounce cans low sodium low fat chicken broth and one cup water to soup pot, two minced cloves of garlic, one chopped onion, one quarter cup of brown rice, one cup corn*. Add one to two pounds of browned in nonfat non stick cooking stray or water, or boiled chicken breasts. Simmer covered or slow cook for 45 minutes or until rice is tender. Add low sodium Italian seasoning and pepper to taste.

* Corn maybe cut from ear, drained from can, or frozen whole kernel corn. Shelled green peas and green beans may be fresh or frozen.

** May substitute one or two pounds of medium shrimp that is cleaned, white fillet fish, or select cut beef in place of chicken. May microwave fish or brown in nonfat no stick cooking spray or water. May boil or brown select cut beef similar to chicken breast.

Dietary Supplements, Food and Liquid Facts, and Helpful Definitions.

1. Beta Carotene: Dietary consumption has shown to increases our immune system, act as an antioxidant by decreasing the risk of lung cancer for smokers. However, it should not be taken as a supplement because it may increase the risk of lung cancer. Found in squash, carrots, and broccoli.

2. Black Tea and Green Tea: Shown to decrease risk for skin and stomach cancer, stroke, and inhibit tooth decay. Milk or other dairy products may inactivate its beneficial effect.

3. Cardiovascular Disease: Buildup of material inside our blood vessels causing a decrease in blood supplied to surrounding tissues. Predominately effects the blood supply to the heart.

4. Cholesterol Profile: Components include Low Density Lipoprotein (LDL), High Density Lipoprotein (HDL), and Triglyceride. The LDL and Triglyceride are the bad cholesterol in that they increase our risk for cardiovascular disease. Our HDL is the good cholesterol in that it is cardio-protecting, and is correlated to our physical activity. In general, if your HDL is below 40 then you are considered sedentary, while above 50 means that your are active.

5. Eggs: Actually low in saturated fatty acids, but high in cholesterol. Saturated fatty acids elevate our LDL level six times greater compared to cholesterol.

6. Fiber: Nondigestible fiver decreases the amount of fatty acids from being absorbed through our digestive lining. Also increases gastrointestinal motility and neutralizes many cholesterol causing a decrease in total cholesterol. Decreases the rate of carbohydrate absorption through our gut lining which prevents large amounts of glucose from hitting our blood stream all at once. Boiling vegetables and beans such as kidney or pinto and then straining them cause a loss in dietary fiber. Recommend twenty to thirty five grams of dietary fiber a day.

7. Garlic: Lowers our LDL cholesterol but may increase Triglycerides. Triglycerides are approximately one fifth as detrimental as LDL. Shown to be an antioxidant and antiviral agent. May also lower blood pressure. Twelve grams of fish oil and 900 milligrams of garlic was shown to lower LDL and Triglyceride levels.

8. Grape Juice: Purple grapes inhibit platelet activity. Recommend one 10 ounce glass per week. Seven 10 ounces glasses are equivalent to aspirins platelet inhibition effects.

9. Homocysteine: High serum levels cause changes in arterial walls which lead to increased rate of cardiovascular disease and is considered an independent risk factor for Cardiovascular Disease. Can be lowered by 650 to 1000 milligrams a day of folic acid or folate as a supplement, preferably in the form of a multivitamin that also contains Thiamine. Folic acid is found in leafy green vegetables, yellow vegetables, meat, poultry, and

enriched grains. The average amount of folate that we consume from our diet is approximately 200 milligrams a day.

10. Iron: Foods containing iron include brown beans, peas, lean meat.

11. Meat temperature. US Department of Agriculture's current recommendations for safely cooked meat so that it is bacteria-free include the following: A. Roast, steak, pork at 145 degrees. B. Egg dishes, casseroles, and ground meat at 150 degrees. C. Left overs 165 degrees. D. Whole chicken, turkey at 180 degrees. Use a meat thermometer and test the temperature in the thickest part of the meat, away from the bone. Checking the meats color or that the juices are clear is not an accurate test.

12. Oats: The dietary fiber associated with it, hs been shown to lower our LDL by blocking saturated fatty acids from being absorbed through our digestive lining. At least one gram of dietary fiber per serving is needed to lower our LDL profile. Saturated fats cause our LDL level to go up.

13. Peanuts: Contain resveratrol which has cardiovascular protecting qualities similar to red wine or aspirin. Loaded with polyunsaturated fats which are considered beneficial to the heart compared to saturated or trans fatty acids.

14. Selenium: 200 micrograms per day supplements. Ten year study found statistically significant lower cancer rates in all cancers. Skin cancer showed no difference. Found in pork, beef, wheat bread, pasta, brazil nuts, lamb. We can have a decrease in risk for

all cancers except skin cancer within five years.

15. Trans Fatty Acids: Found in desserts made with hydrogenated vegetable oil such as cookies, crackers, pastries, and cakes. Also found in margarine, french fries, and many fast food items. Considered the most detrimental of the fatty acids to our heart and blood vessels. A high risk artery clogger, and also associated with an increased risk for breast cancer.

16. Vitamin E: Thought to slow the progression of cardiovascular disease and decrease our risks for cancer. Is a fat soluble vitamin. Not considered beneficial as supplement fo r those of us under 60 years of age. Individuals 64 years and up supplemented with 200 mg per day showed an increase in immune system activity. Higher doses are detrimental. The combination of one gram of vitamin C and 800 IU of vitamin E reduces the damage to our blood vessel caused by foods that are high in fat, if supplemented before the meal.

www.ingramcontent.com/pod-product-compliance
Lightning Source LLC
Chambersburg PA
CBHW060638290526
45793CB00001B/296